Ketogenic Diet:

An Easy Book to Start Your Keto Diet

How to Lose Weight through Rapid Fat Loss

Gain Healthy Body and Unstoppable Energy

Includes the Best Fat Burning Low-Carb Recipes

Table of Contents

Introduction

Oftentimes, engaging in laborious efforts to keep fit and trim becomes exasperating, to the extent that it does not make any sense. Instead of aiming to lose weight, you eventually end up losing your patience! On the one hand, the mélange of weight loss programs passing as fads confuses you even more. On the other hand, coping rigorously with their corresponding guidelines only entails great difficulties, if not, becoming a bore.

As a resolve, this book incisively presents the ketogenic diet to be your ultimate solution. The amazing regimen principally results to shedding your unwanted kilos while allowing yourself to remain fit and keep you on your toes! Lest thinking warily that it has a catch, the diet even tolerates you to eat more fats!

Yes, you have rightly read it: eating fat to keep you fit! If this sounds like science fiction to you, better believe it. It is not a myth, never! Wait until you digest the meat of the matter!

Essentially, the unconventional ketogenic diet is exclusively a high-fat consumption regimen. Butter, vegetable oils, and heavy cream are the diet's usual components to provide the necessary fats. Fats, thereby, give rise to letting you shy away from sweets (glucose-based carbohydrates).

Through replacing simple carbohydrates with healthy fats, the ketogenic diet necessitates your body to be a virtual fat-burning machine! Sooner than you expect, your cognitive process increases while your appetite decreases; thereby, resulting in dramatic weight losses.

Although the regimen strictly restricts various carbohydrate-rich foods, it accepts an even more generous level of tolerances. Nevertheless, meals must be prepared meticulously and measured accordingly.

Certainly, you must have misgivings or doubts about the diet by all its particular food tolerances and restrictions. On the contrary, the perception that fats are bad for your health is fast becoming a yarn. It no longer entails to warn. Medical science and research are helping us improve our understanding of proper nutrition. We have now learned that several types of fats are indeed healthy for our body!

In case you did not know, fats clearly manifest major improvements in several health risk factors, like cholesterol levels. The fact is that the ketogenic diet continuously provides slews of proven health and wellness benefits.

This is the reason why variously new tweaked adaptations of the regimen mushroomed, yet, merely existed as short-lived trends. They capitalized much upon the marketing ploy of losing weight but compromised the essence of staying healthy and fit.

The Atkins or low carbohydrate high fat (LCHF) diet is among the most recognized of these modifications. The only distinction between the two is that the keto diet restricts proteins. At any rate, the ketogenic diet has already long established its basic concept and working principles, and thus, remain to be a proven and efficient weight loss discipline.

Initially, the indulgence of the ketogenic diet was popular for people afflicted with seizures and epilepsy. Nevertheless, no one can really determine its working mechanisms, particularly in controlling seizures. Despite the established theories about how the diet works, the only assurance for treatment is the existence of metabolic changes influencing the chemical composition of the brain.

Hereupon these pages contain your comprehensive guide towards a better understanding of the ketogenic diet. They direct you primarily towards learning about the principle of achieving the ideal metabolic state under optimal ketosis. Furthermore, this book aims to distinguish the ketogenic regimen as an instituted medical nutrition therapy of consuming more fats to lose weight.

The information gained from this book prepares you towards the proper implementation of the diet. Firstly, a definite shopping list of food groups enables you forming prudent decisions on selecting your ideal keto meal; alternatively, desisting certain restricted foods.

Secondly, the book provides you with a dozen of inspiring and delectable keto recipes, grouped into breakfast, desserts and sweets, entrée, salad and side dish, and soup categories. These easy to prepare recipes comprise your 7-day keto meal plan. Exciting as it could be, you will eventually have your shining moment to concoct your own recipes or formulate variations, as soon as you get the hang of practicing your personal ketogenic diet program!

Everything you need to know now is about to unfold on each folio. Upon reaching the book's final canto, bid adieu as a tyro, and emerge as a learned pro about keto! Enjoy reading throughout and keep turning the pages! Along the process, you will earn to learn something priceless! Read on to fruition... to proper nutrition... to weighing less... to good health and wellness!

Chapter 1 – Faith to Eat Fat is Fate to Keep Fit!

Believe it, or not! You need not fast to lose fat! Rather, feast on fats unrestrained, and witness the fastness of fatness gone and fitness gained!

Foremost, this primary chapter aims to help you attain a deeper understanding of the basic concept of the ketogenic diet. It answers why most medical practitioners and health experts consider the diet as most beneficial for you. Not only does the regimen address issues about weight loss or the chemistry of the brain, but also encompass various programs for your health and general welfare.

Roots of the Regimen

Low-carbohydrate intake, fasting, and similar other regimens related to the ketogenic diet have been in existence since ancient times. Mostly, they were common practices for the treatment of epilepsy and neurological disorders.

In 1921, Dr. Rawle Geyelin recorded lesser epileptic and other seizure attacks to all his patients, and the effects had even seemed lasting. Thereafter, Geyelin formulated a more satisfactory diet consisting of a low-carbohydrate and high-fat intake.

While medical practitioners institutionally applied the diet to epileptic patients, the application went into a dramatic decline upon the advent of modern anti-epileptic treatments. Besides, media sensationalized the diet's perceived repute as a starvation regimen.

It was only during the recent past that more and more people renewed their interest towards the diet. This was mainly due to the public's recognition of the persisting medical studies showing proofs about the myriad of health benefits of the ketogenic diet. Currently, medical research and development continue unveiling the diet's mysteries, aside from its original purpose of treating epilepsy.

The French Paradox: An Offshoot to the Keto Diet

The catchphrase, 'French paradox,' sums up the apparent epidemiological notion that the average French incur relatively low incidences of coronary heart disease (CHD); that is, despite indulging a regimen rich in saturated fats. A staple of the noted French diet more often comprises bread, butter, full-fat cheese and yogurt, fresh fruits and vegetables (either grilled or sautéed), wine, small portions of meat (more usually, chicken or fish instead of red meat), and dark chocolate.

Apparently, this observation contradicts the popular belief that such high consumption of fats entails risk factors leading to CHD. Thus, the paradox is that, if the premise associating saturated fats to CHD is well grounded, then the French should have obtained higher frequencies of acquiring CHD compared to nationalities consuming lesser amounts of fats.

Such a paradox is similarly evident vis-à-vis the mechanics of practicing the ketogenic diet, which is essentially a low-carbohydrate, high fat, and moderate protein consumption regimen.

The ketogenic diet derived its name from ketogenesis. It is actually the process of generating ketone bodies, which are intermediate products from the breakdown of fats. This process is a normal alternative function of our body's metabolic processes that allows us to survive without food for longer periods.

Ketogenesis occurs to all of us, especially when we fast, or lower our carbohydrate consumption. This denotes that ketogenesis suppresses your appetite without feeling the gnawing hunger pangs of fasting. Thus, indulging in a diet rich in fats but low in carbohydrates enhances ketogenesis.

That said, you would no longer wonder about the fundamental reason for the French paradox. In the same way, ketogenesis has truly become a doc's paradigm for a disciplinary regimen. Either for longevity or weight loss or even for your general body wellness, you rather engage in the keto diet! Do what the French do! Be part of the French paradox!

While the genesis of the ketogenic diet was for the treatment of epilepsy, ketogenesis has now become a doc's paradigm as a fast way to lose fats to keep fit and healthy!

Chapter 2 – The Amazing Nutritional Switch— Glucose to Fat Metabolism: Working Principle of the Keto Diet

Altering your body function to undergo ketogenesis is altering your life towards health and wellness! Make the big switch, and have your excess weight ditched!

Your main purpose now is how to govern your body into tapping its alternative function of undergoing ketogenesis to generate ketone bodies! This is actually shifting your body's metabolic function from the usual processing of carbohydrates to ketone bodies for the creation of your body's energy.

Curricular Fundamentals of Cellular Fuels

As a review, it is noteworthy that your body cells typically metabolize oxygen and food nutrients during its cellular respiration, or your body's natural dynamics to obtain energy. This metabolic process then creates your principal cellular energy source. Actually, your body cells can avail of two major categories of food-based fuel to create your body's energy:

1. Glucose — Also known as blood sugar, it comes from starches, proteins, and sugars (carbohydrates) in your diet. Although your body requires this cellular fuel system, it is limited. Your body can only store roughly 1,000 to 1,600 calories of glucose. Note that as you perform your regular daily chores, you discharge more or less 2,000 calories.

Therefore, if your body relies solely on sugar to energize itself, your body's energy would certainly drain. Likewise, you exhaust all the stored energy in your body cells if you are not able to feed yourself for more than one day. Clearly, this is not up to, and apt for healthy living.

2. Ketone Bodies — Sourced from fats and produced by fat metabolism, ketones enable your body cells to be functionally flexible. Over time, when your body incurs low glucose levels, your erstwhile glucose-reliant cells automatically switch to using ketone bodies to burn fat for fuel.

Ketone bodies bear unique, yet, favorable characteristics. Compared to glucose, they result to lesser oxidative impairments to your cells. Thus, ketones are safer and healthier fuels for your body cells to use. This also indicates that they function better to generate much more energy than it does from using glucose.

On the average, your body allows storing hundreds of thousands of calories composed of fats. Conclusively, this cellular fuel system simply denotes to having an unlimited energy supply. It now only depends on how long you keep up living through without food.

Metabolism Mechanics

Essentially, the working principle of partaking fats to lose weight is allowing your body to enter ketosis. This results when your body taps the function of ketogenesis. Ketosis is a metabolic state of energy that your body utilizes to supply a substitute fuel when the availability of glucose is low. In short, it is merely switching your body from restricting carbohydrate-rich glucose into a high-fat consumption in order to realize ketosis!

Characteristically, ketosis manifests an abnormal accumulation of ketone bodies. Ketones, like blood sugar, are acidic chemical molecules found in your bloodstream. Your body cells, especially your liver, are the key producers of these ketone bodies for conversion into energy.

The energy production takes place when your body cells break down your body fats. To certain degrees, the physiological energy produced eventually powers up your muscles and body organs. These include important organs like your brain and your entire nervous system.

The production of ketone bodies improves through decreased insulin levels in your bloodstream. When reduced, insulin barely regulates your body's stored fuel (glycogen). At the same time, these pancreatic hormones accelerate oxidation of sugar in your cells. Such bodily cell mechanics is the optimum effect of a low-carbohydrate, low-protein, and high-fat consumption— the ketogenic diet!

Glue Glucose to a Close! Fit Fats as Fuel to Flow Well!

The conclusive determination of achieving optimal ketosis through a regulated low-carb, low protein, and high fat regimen does not necessarily imply that carbohydrates are no longer important. While ketone bodies are beneficial, your body also needs to retain adequate amounts of glucose.

For the most part, glucose is for the requirement purposes of your red blood cells and brain. Nonetheless, when your body abstains from food within extended periods, it forces to break down muscles and fats to produce glucose for the brain.

With the absence of glucose, your brain dies, and so, with your body. This particular glucose requirement for your brain is chiefly the reason why dietitians insist on correcting the false belief that carbohydrates are important nourishments (i.e., we ought to eat them, or else, we die).

Biochemically, this is a faulty declaration. Dietitians fail considering your brain's flexibility of utilizing ketones. In fact, this metabolic process ably produces more than half of the glucose that your brain demands. More importantly, it occurs as soon as your body becomes keto-adapted (efficient at burning ketones for fuel).

As a conclusion, glucose may be essential for your brain; yet, consuming carbohydrates to create glucose is NOT, particularly, if you are undergoing ketosis. In short, shifting from a carbohydrate-derived diet to a dietary fat-based regimen should be your preferred body fuel!

The switch helps greatly towards rebalancing your body's chemistry. It entails a positively natural effect of weight loss. Additionally, it includes better weight management upon reaching your ideal weight. This explains why you do not really get fat from exercising less and eating much. Neither do you get fat from consuming fat.

Essentially, overeating or obesity can be a perception of symptoms of an inappropriate diet. These severe cases are not necessarily the causes of consuming calories abundantly per se. Instead, these are results of acquiring calories from wrongful sources. Besides, other factors cause obesity or excessive body weight.

Misconceptions and Misinterpretations

It has been a common misconception that the ketogenic diet is likely expensive. As it could be obvious to low-carbohydrate diets, you perceive and estimate the high costs of meat. On the contrary, this is an erroneous perspective since the ketogenic diet focuses moderately on proteins and more on fats that allow you to save more by emphasizing primarily on the fats.

Ketosis may connote impressions in various forms. It can be a case of either Type-I diabetes mellitus or alcoholism or starvation. It is a condition wherein the fat-burning rate of your body is extremely high. During this state, ketones in your blood begin increasing.

However, do not mistake ketosis with the grave condition of ketoacidosis (lack of insulin and abnormally high acidity of the blood). Ketosis is actually nutritional. Ergo, it is a normally safe human condition!

Nevertheless, an excessive accumulation of ketones can heighten the acidity of your blood. In most cases, this results in some critical issues. When left neglected or unchecked, ketosis can severely affect your urine. Certain urine infections may lead to either serious liver or kidney failure. Thus, it is apparent that fasting is an outright ill-advised idea.

Also, since ketosis may associate itself to starvation, do not confuse the ketogenic diet as a form of intermittent fasting. This is completely a different, yet an extreme disciplinary regimen.

Therefore, be careful as you plan to start practicing the regimen. It is necessary to place yourself under close supervision by your medical adviser. When performed properly and responsibly, the ketogenic diet can be an effective treatment for several health problems.

Achieving Optimal Ketosis is A-OK!

Oftentimes, several adherents to the strict keto diet become wary that ketone levels in their blood fall beyond the ideal figures. This must not come as a surprise to you. The key to practicing the regimen properly is avoiding all foods derived from carbohydrates. You must be restrictive on your carbohydrates consumption, which must only allow you less than 15g daily. Getting quickly into a state of ketosis depends on your food consumption

More so, you should also be cautious with your protein intakes. Consuming substantial quantities of protein causes your body to convert the excesses into glucose. Besides, large protein consumptions increase insulin levels. As a result, this compromises your goal of attaining optimal ketosis. To address such a dilemma, it is highly advisable to satisfy your cravings with more fats. As queer as it may seem, this peculiar advice certainly weaves wonders for you.

In principle, ingesting more fats allows you to feel fuller. It abruptly suppresses taking further food servings and ensures lesser intakes of carbohydrates and proteins. In the process, a high-fat regimen directly addresses your excess weight issues. Definitely, insulin levels drop; and thereby, your body achieves optimal ketosis.

To maximize your results under the ketogenic diet, achieve undergoing optimal ketosis. However, this is not recommendable for individuals who have Type-1 diabetes. The trick here is to not only restrict you from partaking carbohydrates but also be aware of your protein intake. The secret, unbelievably, is having your fill with lots of fats!

Keystone Labels of Ketone Levels

As previously stated, the overproduction of ketone bodies increases your blood's acidity that leads to further health complications. Thus, it is only proper to check and measure your ketone levels. The ideal way of measuring ketones is on an empty stomach. Preferably, perform your measurements before breakfast.

Ketone bodies manifest in your urine. You may apply the traditional spot test of using chemically coated dipsticks, available from pharmacies. However, these do not give you accurate measurements, leaving you clueless on the exact presence and concentration of ketones.

The more innovative and pricey gadgets are more reliable for accurate measurements. Although most devices require pricking your finger with a needle, you can readily determine your blood ketone levels precisely within seconds.

The succeeding labeled parameters are your guidelines to interpret variously ranged values of ketone levels measured in millimoles per liter (mmol/L):

Less than 0.50-mmol/L — signifies a ketone count that is far beyond optimum levels of fat burning. This shows that your body is not in a state of ketosis. Thus, it only indicates having normal levels of ketones.

Within 0.50 to 1.50-mmol/L — denotes a moderate ketone count that results in a better weight reduction and fat metabolism with no insulin deficiency. However, this does not show optimum conditions of ketosis. Rather, this portrays that your body is only undergoing light nutritional ketosis.

Within 1.50 to 3.0-mmol/L — demonstrates the recommended ketone levels for maximum weight loss. This exhibits the ideal state of attaining optimum ketosis. Nevertheless, watch out when reaching the verge of higher ketone levels. The chances are that you may be at risk for diabetic ketoacidosis. Contact your doc immediately for further advice.

More than 3.0-mmol/L — connotes neither achieving better nor worse conditions compared to ketone levels within 1.5-3 mmol/L. Thus, ketone counts falling under this range are negligible values. Sometimes, higher ketone levels depict your body as having lower food intake. It only means that you are undergoing a serious metabolic condition, and a prompt medical care is indeed necessary.

You do not get fat as such from exercising less and eating much!

Neither do you get fat from consuming fat!

The secret is attaining ketosis... impose a fatty dose as you dispose glucose!

Chapter 3 – Proper Program Performance

Whatever you do, you do it well! If not, better bid farewell!

Have the discipline and determination to satisfy your expectation!

The keto regimen, like any other training or discipline,

its difficulties are just always at the beginning!

With frequency, it would simply be as easy as counting 123... and reciting your ABC!

Fundamentally, the ketogenic diet is a medical nutrition therapy. It crucially involves participants from various medical disciplines. The team may include a neurologist, experienced in prescribing the ketogenic diet; a certified nurse, knowledgeable enough with the cause and effects of the diet; and, a licensed dietitian, coordinating with the regular program of the diet.

Furthermore, additional assistance may come from a registered pharmacist, advising upon certain dosages of prescribed medicines and carbohydrate values, and a certified medical social practitioner working together with the family. Lastly, for its safe and proper implementation, other caregivers, as well as immediate family members must have the necessary understanding of the various aspects of the regimen.

Upon planning to practice the keto diet, heed the advice of availing the close supervision from your medical adviser. Somehow, there are risks of complicating matters during the program's initiation. For example, if you have acquired Type-1 diabetes mellitus, never proceed to achieve optimal ketosis since it may pose further harm on your health. Nonetheless, if ketones are truly present in your blood, always ensure that your blood sugar must be at normal levels.

A normal blood sugar level denotes to be at normal ketosis, just like the ketosis exhibited by healthy individuals practicing a strict low-carbohydrate diet. On the contrary, a high blood sugar level with high ketones only demonstrates that insulin levels are pathologically low.

While non-diabetics do not actually suffer from these risky levels, this may result in diabetes acidosis, or ketoacidosis, which could be a life-threatening case. If such condition occurs, the body needs more insulin injections. Nevertheless, prudence always dictates that you ought to seek medical advice when you are never sure at all. Gaining high ketone levels for losing weight is never worth the risk for people with Type-1 diabetes.

Regimen's Rules

It is inevitable that the performance of the keto diet eventually takes many forms. Yet, its standard practice consists typically of daily carbohydrate restrictions not more than 50 grams. While wanting to keep your carbohydrates restricted, your inclination of food consumption must principally derive from dairy, nuts, and vegetables. Mostly, your meals must comprise proteins with vegetables, including ample amounts of healthy fats. (Refer to Chapter 4).

More importantly, it is ideal following the formulaic 60-35-5 nutritional value proportion, wherein, 60% of all calories come from fats, 35% from proteins, and 5% from carbohydrates. Proteins should be set between 1.5g to 1.75g per kilogram of your ideal body weight. High-protein consumptions prevent your body from undergoing optimal ketosis.

Now, for clearer comparisons, an average Westerner's diet comprises about 65 to 85% of carbohydrates, 10 to 20 % of fats, and 5 to 15% of proteins! By Jove, that is completely an exact opposite! Anyway, that is what usually happens, especially when one is, used to expending body energy sourced from carbohydrate-based foods; if not, possessing the wrong notions of fearing to eat fats!

Nevertheless, meals should be meticulously prepared, as well as measured accordingly on a gram scale. The standard ketogenic diet comprises usual of ratios (in grams) of carbohydrates to protein ratios of 3:1 and 4:1.

Understanding and Using the Rated Ratio

An important part of leading a healthy and fit lifestyle is exercise. By exercising, it necessarily involves a recovery phase and caring for your body. This stage can be unique to each individual, considering the types and extents of exercises one may perform. Recovering fittingly in the healthiest means possible is merely following a basic carb to protein ratio.

The carb to protein ratio is actually the amount of carbohydrates relative to the amount or proteins you take. While the keto diet may entail several ratios to follow, they are generally dependent upon the intensity of the performed exercises or activities. The 4 to 1 ratio is normally more suitable for more intense workouts. For those inclined on non-endurance cardio programs or moderate weights lifting, it is considerable to implement either a 2 to 1 or 3 to 1 ratio.

4:1 Ratio Creation

For purposes of convenience and simplicity after your workout, you can readily grab from among the several energy recovery snacks available that already have the formulated 4:1 ratio you need.

Still, you have all the liberty of choosing to formulate your own ratio. The following will serve as your example guide of food combinations, which ensure your body will be receiving what it adequately needs.

Simply combining each list of ingredients together will also give you the necessary 4:1 carbohydrate to protein ratio:

- Apple or orange, and almonds

- Apple or orange, and string cheese

- Banana, cheese, and whole-grain crackers

- Hummus and whole-wheat pitas

- Milk and oats or oatmeal

- Nonfat plain Greek yogurt, honey, and blueberries

For example, you chose to use combining nonfat plain Greek yogurt, honey, and blueberries. Your principal protein source then is yogurt. As you will check to see the amount in grams of protein per serving, Greek yogurt has 18g of proteins per 100-calorie serving (6oz.). Thus, this denotes that you need a total of 72g of carbohydrates (18 × 4) for this food combo to achieve your 4:1 ratio.

Therefore, with 2-Tbsp of honey having 34g of carbs, plus 1-½ cups of blueberries having 31g of carbs, and Greek yogurt having 7g of carbs, the summation of carbohydrates amounts to 72 grams! For this example, the total calories— 100 calories of yogurt, plus 126 calories of blueberries plus 128 calories of honey— will be 354 calories at a ratio of 4:1.

As the case may be, you can just adjust the amounts accordingly so that they may be within what suits your purposes. Note that this is just only for intense workouts. Obviously, you do not want to be exercising and burning 200 calories, and thereafter, grabbing for a 4:1 and 354-calorie snack.

The rule of thumb is using only the 4:1 ratio for intense exercise; eat approximately half of your workout calorie; and, burn in your post-workout your 4:1 snack. Hence, if you burn 600 calories in an intense workout, you should eat about 300 calories thereafter. If you had a brief workout and only burned 400 calories, then you ought to adjust to a 200-calorie snack.

ADDENDUM: Implementing the keto diet may baffle caregivers, patients or practitioners alike with difficulties, mainly due to the time spent and devoted to planning and measuring the meals. Yet, as it should always be the case, any unplanned meals have the possibilities of breaking momentum on the regular necessities of nutritional balance.

For the diet's optimum efficiency, consume your measured food in its entirety!

Plan before you use! Apply the ratios; conform to the values!

Chapter 4 – Regimen's Regulated Rations

You can enjoy eating almost everything by practicing the diet!

There are somehow a few restrictions to set; yet, you can really cope and live with it, you bet!

Indulging in any dietary program is never the easiest and comfortable thing in the world to perform, particularly when you are unaware or unsure about what you ought to consume or eat. This whole chapter presents together the recommended and restricted food list of the ketogenic diet to guide you in making prudent decisions about what you should be consuming and/or including in your grocery list.

Recommended Rations

When you are about to get started on a ketogenic diet, you must know about the following food list below, which comprises the most noted high-fat and low-carbohydrate foods. The list, outlined and categorized under major food groups, is by no means encompassing in scope. At any rate, it directs you properly towards the right direction and helps you to stay on course.

Proteins

You should be extra cautious about the quantities of protein you consume over time, since your body may eventually adapt the process of gluconeogenesis— the conversion of proteins into glucose. That is far from your purpose!

Hence, you should test to check whether your consumption of protein is hindering you to attain ketosis. Promptly make the necessary adjustments accordingly. Your best option of protein choices should be anything organic, or grass-fed livestock, aquamarine, and poultry produce. Obviously, organic products entail reduced risks of consuming bacteria and steroid hormones.

For deli meats, go for bologna, ham, sausage, bacon, and salami; cold cuts, like pastrami and turkey breast; pepperoni slices or sticks; and, prosciutto or salt-cured ham. For meats and poultry, go for beef or pork (loins, ribs, ground, chops, steaks, roasts and tips) and chicken or turkey (either whole or parts or ground). For other miscellaneous meat products, opt for beef jerky or beef sticks, and pork rind (crushed, which is a better alternative for breadcrumbs).

Carbohydrates

The quantities of consuming carbohydrates are what exclusively determine a diet as ketogenic. That also includes one's own levels of activity and body metabolism. Normally, it is considerably ketogenic if the diet has a daily composition of not more than 50 to 60 grams of net or effective carbohydrates.

Nonetheless, individuals having healthy body metabolisms can consume more than 100 grams of net carbohydrates daily, yet, retain effective levels of ketosis. Moreover, older people affected with Type-2 diabetes mellitus can only consume less than 30 grams of net carbohydrates daily to achieve similar levels.

Fats and Oils

Fats and oils are the major sources of the ketogenic diet's daily calorie intake. You may combine them in several ways in your meals, in either sauces or dressings or simply placing butter over cooked meat. Although fats are essential to the body, they may also be risky if we eat the wrong types of fats.

The more preferred fats are those monounsaturated and saturated types, which are both chemically stable, yet, less inflammatory to most people such as, coconut oil, butter, avocado, macadamia nuts and egg yolks.

Shun away from hydrogenated lards, like margarine, to minimize consumption of trans-unsaturated fats. In any case, medical studies linked these fats to higher risks of coronary heart diseases. If you use vegetable oils such as safflower or soybean, olives, and flax, always opt for those cold- pressed types.

Therefore, choose non-hydrogenated fats at all times like coconut oil, ghee liquid butter, or beef tallow. Such fats entail higher smoke points, and lesser oxidation compared to other oils, and thus, provide more essential fatty acids. Be cautious though about consuming nut- or seed-based oils such as flaxseed oil, almond oil, and sesame oil. These oils have high contents of inflammatory Omega-6.

Dairy Products

Preferably, dairy food sources of the ketogenic diet should be raw and organic. These include butter; cheese (hard) like parmesan and cheddar; cheese (soft) like Farmer's and Muenster; cream cheese; eggs; full-fat or nonfat plain Greek yogurts, with carbohydrate counts of not more than seven per serving; heavy cream; and, sour cream.

Nuts and Seeds

The ketogenic diet does not prohibit any type of nuts and seeds. They actually work best for the diet, particularly when roasted to extract their anti-nutrient components. However, some of these nuts and seeds are positively high in Omega-6 fatty acids.

Thus, it is only necessary to monitor carefully and have a proper balance when consuming nuts with higher carbohydrate counts like cashews, chestnuts, and pistachios. Regarding carbohydrate values, macadamias, almonds, hazelnuts, pecans, and walnuts are ideal.

Furthermore, nut and seed flours such as almond flour and milled flax seed can be excellent alternatives to regular flour. Sunflower, pumpkin, and sesame are the most preferred seeds to use with the diet.

Sugar Substitutes and Sweeteners

You are definitely on the safe side when abstaining yourself from anything sweet. Over time, the abstention inclines you to curtail your sweet tooth cravings. If it is inevitable for you to lust for something sweet, then, better favor artificial sweeteners.

Opt for those liquid sweeteners instead since these do not have extra binders or additives like dextrose and maltodextrin (a carbohydrate with polysaccharides or multiple sugar molecules). Also, good choices are sugar alcohols like Erythritol and Xylitol, and other artificial sweeteners like Splenda® and Swerve®.

Vegetables

Vegetables are extremely significant in any composition for a healthy diet. Nonetheless, certain vegetables do not suit nutritionally in a keto diet due to their high sugar contents or glycemic index (commonly abbreviated as GI, which is a nutritional tool that helps you rate the quality of carbohydrates that you eat).

The best vegetables for a ketogenic diet are those planted above ground and organically grown. Although both organic and non-organic vegetables possess similar nutritional properties and values, organically grown vegetables are more favorable to avoid pesticide and chemical fertilizer residues.

Typically, they are dark and leafy greens, which are rich in nutrients and low in carbohydrates. Examples of such are bell peppers, broccoli, Brussels sprouts, cabbage, cauliflower, cucumber, garlic, kale, lettuce, okra, onion, spinach, squash, and zucchini.

Herbs and Spices

This particular food group can be critical in ketogenic foods. Some herbs and spices contain more and heavier carbohydrates than others do such as, bay leaves, allspice, cardamom, cinnamon, ginger, garlic powder, and onion powder. Moreover, ready-made spice mixes have sugars added in them. Thus, it is wise to note their nutrition labels and values.

When using salt, better make use of sea salt instead of table salt. The former is more natural as it retains the trace elements found in saline water while the latter usually contains sugar additives like powdered dextrose (a compound of glucose).

Cooking Condiments/Pantry Particulars

Below is a comprehensive shopping list that serves as your quick grocery guide in selecting the appropriate cooking ingredients for your ketogenic food recipes:

- Bouillon or seasoned broth (chicken or vegetable)

- Canned processed meats (luncheon meat, Vienna sausage)

- Canned seafood (anchovies, crab, salmon, sardines, tuna in oil or water)

- Canned vegetables (hearts of palm, artichoke hearts, green chilies, chipotle peppers, roasted red peppers, mushrooms, and sun-dried tomatoes in oil)

- Cocoa powder (unsweetened)

- Dill pickles or sauerkraut (sugar-free, for salads)

- Extracts— vanilla, lemon, almond, etc. (sugar-free)

- Extra-virgin olive oil

- Flour substitutes (use almond flour or other nut flours)

- Gelatin (plain)

- Horseradish seasoning

- Lemon or lime juice (1 gram of carbohydrate per tablespoon)

- Mayonnaise (choose brands with the lowest carbohydrate content)

- Mustard (except sweetened mustards like honey mustard)

- Nut butter (natural or unsweetened)

- Pickled flower buds or capers

- Salad dressings (sugar-free)

- Salsas and hot sauces (like sriracha, sambal oelek, Tabasco®)

- Sauces (Alfredo's, pasta, and pizza, sugar-free and no thickeners)

- Sesame oil for salad dressings

- Tamari soy sauce (avoid soy sauce if you are gluten intolerant)

- Tomato products (canned tomato paste and tomatoes)

- Whey protein powder (plain, vanilla and chocolate flavors)

- Wine or cider vinegar (use balsamic vinegar sparingly)

- Xanthan gum (for thickening and binding)

Fruits

Fruit consumptions can be optional since they are dependent upon one's health stability and weight conditions. Some people are fructose intolerant while others remain trim and fit despite eating several fruits.

If you indulge partaking fruits, seek fresh fruits in season, and go for those typical fruits with low-sugar content like avocados, grapefruits, olives, and berries. Better, eat fresh fruits combined with a fat component like cheese, whipped cream, or peanut butter. In this manner, it retards sudden rise of your blood sugar levels.

Seafood

Any seafood staple is always a healthy diet. The best options would include fresh or frozen salmons, tunas, scallops, and shrimps, or any type of aquamarine produce farmed or caught in the wild. Such sea produce contains healthy fish oils or higher fat levels of polyunsaturated fatty acids (PUFA) Omega-3.

Beverages

Practicing the keto diet creates a natural diuretic effect; so, dehydration is a common occurrence. Thus, you should be ready to take plenty of liquids to keep yourself hydrated, no matter if you have a urinary tract infection or being prone to bladder pains. However, be cautious with liquids that contain sweeteners since they may consist of carbohydrates.

Regimen's Restricted Rations

Somehow, it becomes inevitable at times to include unknowingly certain foods that do not really belong to your ketogenic dietary program. Just because you only perceived such foods supposedly compose of high fat and low carbohydrate contents, it does not mean that they are outright significant contributors towards the diet's requirements. This should never be the case.

Therefore, to help you properly identify further which should be which, hereunder is a list of foods that you must be more wary about their inclusion in your ketogenic diet:

Tomato Derivatives—are essentially abundant in sugar— especially when processed like packed tomato sauces and canned diced tomatoes— despite noted universally as healthy foods. Hence, know your required portions by their nutritional labels. In certain cases, food companies cunningly mislead you with the nutritional values of serving sizes to let their products appear healthier.

As a rule, avoid processed and canned foods when you can. Obviously, you are always unsure of their origins, derivations, and compositions, not to mention their unhealthy and diminished nutritional values.

Diet Soda – are indispensable liquids for hydrating purposes; thus, the ketogenic diet does not actually disallow you from drinking it. Instead, always be conscious with your drinking quantities since they correspond proportionally to intakes of artificial sweeteners.

Peppers – unbelievably contain sugars no matter how pungent and hot they are. Be on the lookout for these seasonings in chili-based food preparations. Rather choose green peppers, since both those red and yellow varieties contain higher carbohydrate contents.

Fruits – possess high sugar contents in the form of fructose. Generally, the keto diet excludes fruits. Nevertheless, it is still possible to eat them for as long as you follow their allowable serving sizes strictly.

Medicine – either branded over-the-counter or generic drugs such as cough syrups, colds, and flu medications, usually contain carbohydrates in great amounts. Be on your guard about these medicines. For your information, there are several alternative drugs available that have a lower sugar content, if not, completely sugar-free.

As a summary, it is a wise advice to adhere to eating mostly natural, unprocessed, organic, and fresh foods. Although processed or canned foods can be beneficial and convenient as grab-and-go foods, or when you wish to take anything instantly with low carbohydrate contents, consuming foods in their most natural form is always much cleaner and healthier.

Preparing and dining on a keto meal can be tricky!

Essentially, it only demands for an appropriate recipe!

The technique is taking everything in regulation... and, knowing what is best for your consumption!

Chapter 5 – Breakfast Recipes

1. Spinach, Sausage, and Feta Frittata

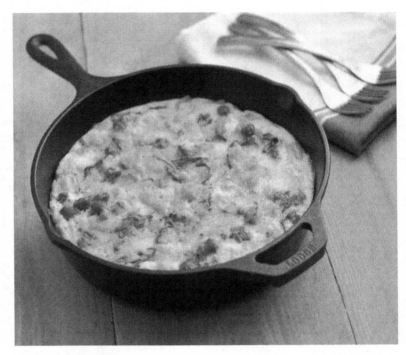

Ingredients:

12-oz sausage, sliced into small pieces

12-pcs eggs

10-oz pack frozen chopped spinach, thawed, drained, and squeezed dry

½-cup Feta cheese, crumbled

½-cup heavy cream

½-cup almond milk, unsweetened

½-tsp salt

¼-tsp black pepper

¼-tsp ground nutmeg

Directions:

In a medium-sized bowl, place the sliced raw sausages. Break the spinach up into the same bowl as the sausage.

Sprinkle Feta cheese over the mixture. Toss lightly until fully combined. Spread the mixture lightly onto a greased casserole.

In a larger bowl, combine the beaten the eggs with almond milk, nutmeg, cream, salt, and pepper together. Mix thoroughly until blended well.

Pour the mixture gently into the casserole for about ¾ full.

Bake at 375ºF for 50 minutes until fully set. Serve warm or at room temperature.

Yield: 12-triangular slices

Nutritional values per serving: 206 Calories | 16g Fat | 1.4g Net Carbohydrates | 12g Protein

2. Cream Cheese Pancake

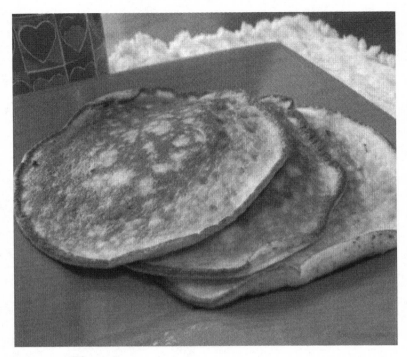

Ingredients:

2-pcs eggs

2-oz cream cheese

1-packet sweetener

½-tsp cinnamon

Directions:

In a blender, combine all ingredients, and blend until smooth. Let it stand for 2 minutes for the bubbles to settle.

Grease a hot pan with butter. Pour a fourth of the batter into the pan. Cook for about 2 minutes until golden. Flip and cook 1 minute on the other side.

Repeat the procedure with the remaining batter. Serve with sugar-free syrup and fresh berries of choice.

Yield: 4 x 6-inch diameter pancakes

Nutritional values per serving: 344 Calories | 29g Fat | 2.5g Net Carbohydrates | 17g Protein

3. Scrambled Eggs with Mayonnaise

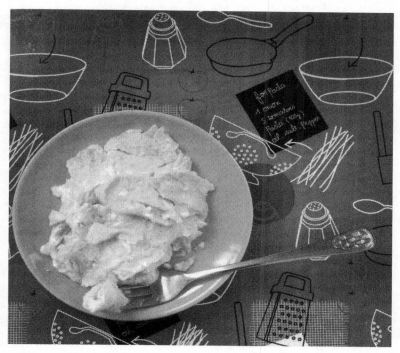

Ingredients:

50g raw egg

23g mayonnaise (organic)

10g butter

Directions:

Melt butter in a non-stick pan. In the meantime, mix the egg and mayonnaise together until fully combined.

Pour the egg and mayo mixture into the pan; cook until set. Scrape the eggs and all the remaining fat onto a serving plate and serve immediately.

Yield: one serving

Nutritional values per serving: 308 Calories | 31.27g Fat | 0.53g Net Carbohydrates | 6.38g Protein

Chapter 6 – Entrée Recipes

1. Rib-eye Steak

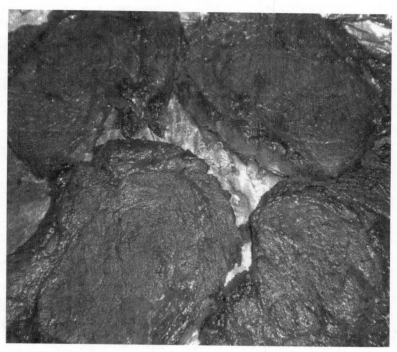

Ingredients:

1-16oz rib-eye steak (1 to 1¼-inch thick)

1-tbsp   duck fat (or peanut oil)

1-tbsp butter

½-tsp thyme, chopped

Salt and pepper to taste

Directions:

Preheat oven to 400°F and place a cast iron skillet inside.

Prepare the rib-eye steak by seasoning with oil, salt, and pepper.

Remove the preheated skillet from the oven and set over medium heat. Add oil, and place the steak. Sear for a couple of minutes on both sides.

Place the steak in the oven to roast for about 4 to 6 minutes.

Remove steak and place over the stove, set over low heat.

Add butter and thyme in the skillet, and baste steak for about 2 to 4 minutes.

Let it sit for about 5 minutes, and serve.

Yield: 2-servings

Nutritional values per serving: 750 Calories | 66g Fats | 0g Net Carbohydrates | 38g Protein

2. Spicy Chicken Meatballs

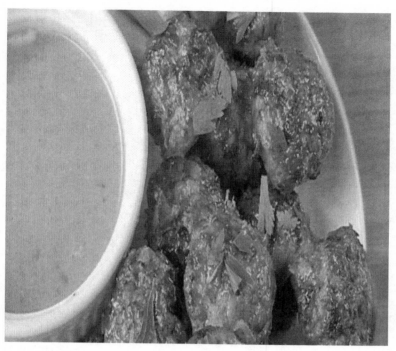

Ingredients:

For the meatballs

2-tbsps flaxseed meal

2-tbsps cilantro, chopped

2-tbsps almond flour

2-pcs spring onions, medium, chopped

2-oz cheddar cheese

1-lb chicken meat, ground

½-tsp salt

½-tsp red pepper flakes

½-tsp garlic powder

½-pc red bell pepper, medium, chopped

Juice and zest of ½-lime, medium

For the guacamole dressing

1-pc avocado, medium

¼-tsp garlic powder

Salt & pepper to taste

Juice of ½-lime, medium

Directions:

For the meatballs

Preheat oven to 350°F. In the meantime, melt the cheddar cheese in the microwave in 20-second intervals until bubbling. Set aside in a bowl.

Add all the ingredients in the bowl of melted cheese. Mix until evenly combined.

Roll the chicken mixture into meatballs uniformly. Bake the chicken meatballs for about 15 to 18 minutes. Set aside after cooking.

For the guacamole dressing

Mash the avocado. Combine the mashed avocado with garlic powder, lime juice, and salt and pepper to taste. Mix well to a smooth consistency.

Serve the chicken meatballs along with the guacamole dressing.

Yield: 3-servings

Nutritional values per serving: 428 Calories | 31.3g Fats | 4.7g Net Carbohydrates | 33.7g Protein

3. Nasi Lemak (Malaysian National Dish)

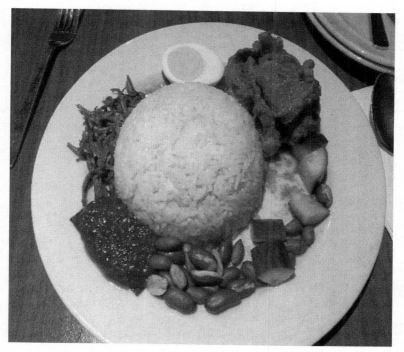

Ingredients:

For the fried chicken

2-pcs chicken thighs, boneless

½-tsp curry powder

¼-tsp turmeric powder

½-tsp lime juice

⅛-tsp salt

½-tsp coconut oil

For the Nasi Lemak

7-oz cauliflower, drained, squeezed dry and sieved in the consistency of rice

5-quarter slices cucumber

3-tbsps coconut milk

3-slices ginger

½-bulb shallot, small

¼-tsp salt, to taste

For the egg

1-pc egg, large

½-tbsp unsalted butter

Directions:

For the fried chicken

Marinate the chicken thighs with lime juice, turmeric powder, curry powder, and salt. Let it stand for 30 minutes.

Fry the marinated chicken thighs. Set aside after cooking.

For the Nasi Lemak

Combine coconut milk, ginger, and shallot in a saucepan, and bring to a boil.

Add the cauliflower, and mix thoroughly. Set aside after cooking.

For the egg

You can either fry or boil the egg. Set aside after cooking.

Arrange the Nasi Lemak and fried chicken over two dishes and serve with slices of cucumber and the fried egg on the side. If desired, add anchovies, peanuts, and sambal oelek or ground red-hot Thai chilies along with the dish.

Yield: 2-servings

Nutritional values per serving: 501.7 Calories | 39.9g Fats | 6.9g Net Carbohydrates | 28.1g Protein

Chapter 7 – Desserts and Sweets Recipes

1. Coconut Candy

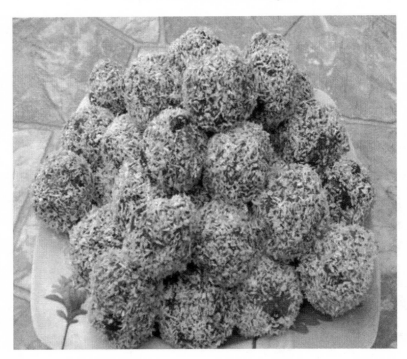

Ingredient

Coconut Butter (or popularly known as Coconut Manna)

Directions

Melt the coconut butter until it resembles a creamy peanut butter consistency.

Spoon out into candy molds. Refrigerate for at least 10 minutes to harden before serving. (You can refrigerate it for several weeks in a closed container.)

Nutritional values per 15g of coconut butter: 102 calories | 10.3gm fat | 1.14g net carbohydrates | 1.14g protein

2. Irish Philadelphia Potato Candy

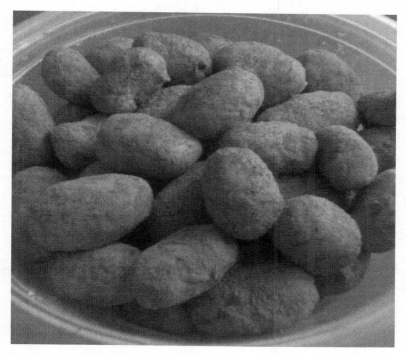

Ingredients

69-g Philadelphia Cream Cheese

16-g shredded coconut, unsweetened

7-g butter, at room temperature

2-g ground cinnamon

Sweetener of choice

Directions

In a bowl, combine all the ingredients except for the cinnamon. Place the mixture in the refrigerator, and allow setting until it hardens.

Apportion the batter by weight by summing up the weight of ingredients less that of the cinnamon, and dividing by number of servings desired.

Roll the portions into potato shapes and place on a sheet of parchment paper. Sprinkle them with cinnamon all over, and store in the refrigerator for a week.

Yield: Eight 50-calorie servings

Nutritional values for entire batch: 401 calories | 40.85g fat | 3.57g net carbohydrates | 6.45g protein

3. Avocado Vanilla Pudding

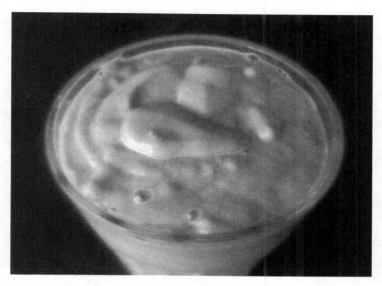

Ingredients

2-ripe Hass avocados, peeled, pitted and cut into chunks

2-teaspoons organic vanilla extract

1 (13.5 fl oz = 400 ml)-can organic coconut milk

1-tablespoon lime juice from organic lime, freshly squeezed

80-drops of liquid stevia

Directions

Combine all the ingredients in a blender, and blend until smooth and velvety.

Yield: Three servings

Nutritional values per serving: 593 calories | 58.3g fat | 3.9g net carbohydrates | 1g protein

Chapter 8 – Salad & Side Dish Recipes

1. Sichuan Shirataki & Cucumber Salad

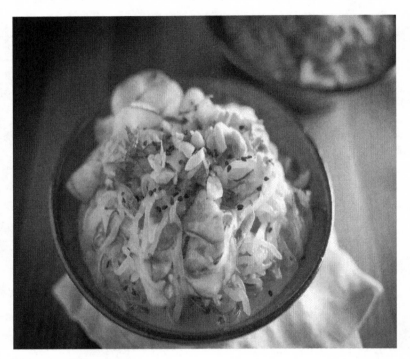

Ingredients:

2-tbsps coconut oil

1-tsp sesame seeds

1-tbsp sesame oil

1-tbsp rice vinegar

1-stalk spring onion, medium

1-packet Sichuan shirataki noodles, rinsed and dried

¾-pc cucumber, large, sliced thinly

¼-tsp red pepper flakes

Salt and pepper to taste

Directions:

Heat the coconut oil in a pan, set over medium-high heat. Add in the dried noodles, and allow frying for 5 to 7 minutes, or until crisp and browned.

After frying, place the noodles on paper towels to cool and dry.

Arrange the sliced cucumber on a plate as to your preference. Place the shirataki noodles over the cucumbers, and top it with red pepper flakes, spring onion, rice vinegar, sesame seeds, sesame oil, and salt and pepper to taste.

Store the dish in the refrigerator for at least half an hour prior to serving.

Yield: One serving

Nutritional values per serving: 416 Calories | 43g Fats | 7g Net Carbohydrates | 2g Protein

2. Spicy Roasted Lemony Broccoli

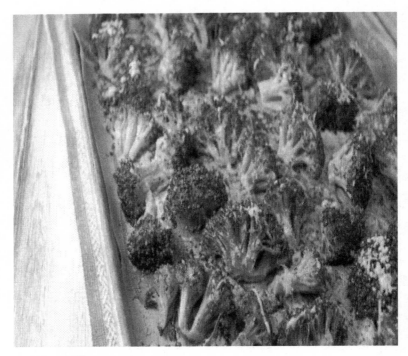

Ingredients:

3-tsps garlic, minced

2-tbsps fresh basil, chopped

1½-lbs broccoli florets

½-tsp red chili flakes

½ to ¾-tsp kosher salt

⅓-cup parmesan cheese

¼-cup olive oil

Zest of ½-pc lemon

Juice of ½-pc lemon

Directions:

Preheat the oven to 425°F.

Arrange broccoli florets on a baking sheet covered with parchment paper.

Season the broccoli with olive oil, chopped fresh basil, minced garlic, kosher salt, red chili flakes, zest and juice of half a lemon each.

Sprinkle parmesan cheese over the top of the broccoli and place in the oven to bake for about 20 to 25 minutes.

Yield: 6-servings

Nutritional values per serving: 137 Calories | 10.5g Fats | 3.7g Net Carbohydrates | 5.7g Protein

3. Brussels Sprouts Fries

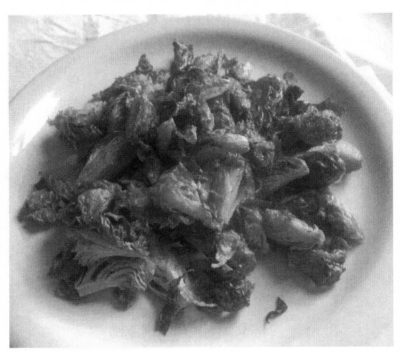

Ingredients:

½-bag Brussels sprouts

2-tbsp parmesan cheese

Salt and pepper to taste

Oil for deep-frying

Directions:

Heat the oil in a deep-fat fryer. Place the Brussels sprouts in the fryer without overcrowding.

Fry the sprouts until browned on the edges of the bulb, and dark green on the leaves.

After frying, place the fries on paper towels to drain excess grease. Sprinkle salt, pepper, and parmesan cheese.

Yield: 2-servings

Nutritional values per serving: 109 Calories | 8.5g Fats | 1.5g Net Carbohydrates | 4g Protein

Chapter 9 – Soup and Puree Recipes

1. Sausage and Pepper Soup

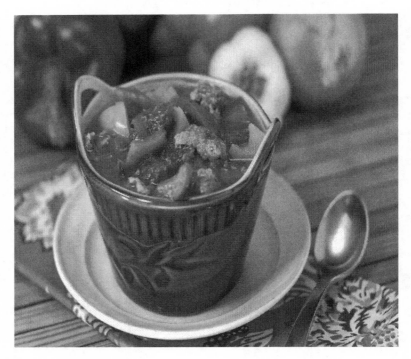

Ingredients:

4-cups beef stock

32-oz pork sausage

1-tsp onion powder

1-tsp Italian seasoning

1-tsp garlic powder

1-tbsp olive oil

1-tbsp cumin

1-tbsp chili powder

1-pc green bell pepper, medium, sliced

1-can tomatoes with jalapenos

10-oz spinach, raw

¾-tsp kosher salt

Directions:

In a large pot over medium-high heat, cook sausage with olive oil until seared. Stir, and cook further.

Add green peppers to the pot, stir well, and season with salt and pepper to taste; add the tomatoes with jalapenos, and stir again; and then, place the spinach on top of and cover the pot with its lid. As the spinach begins to wilt, add the beef broth, spices, and seasonings. Mix well, and cover with its lid again

Cook further for half an hour, while reducing the heat to medium-low.

Take out the pot, cover and allow simmering for 15 minutes. Serve hot.

Yield: 6-servings

Nutritional values per serving: 526 Calories | 43g Fats | 3.8g Net Carbohydrates | 27.8g Protein

2. Pork Stew: Southwestern Style

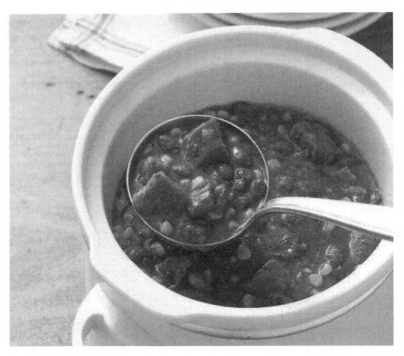

Ingredients:

1-lb cooked pork shoulder, sliced

6-oz button mushrooms

2-tsps chili powder

2-tsps   cumin

2-pcs bay leafs

2-cups gelatinous bone broth

2-cups chicken broth

1-tsp paprika

1-tsp oregano

1-tsp garlic, minced

½-tsp salt

½-tsp pepper

½-pc red bell pepper, sliced

½-pc jalapeno, sliced

½-pc green bell pepper, sliced

½-cup strong coffee

½-bulb onion, medium

¼-tsp cinnamon

¼-cup tomato paste

Juice of ½-lime (to finish)

Directions:

In a pan set over high heat, sauté all the vegetables with olive oil. Remove from the heat once the vegetables exude their aroma.

In a slow cooker, place the sliced pork, together with the gelatinous bone broth, button mushrooms, chicken broth, and strong coffee.

Place the sautéed vegetables and spices in the slow cooker, and mix well. Cover the slow cooker with its lid and allow cooking under low heat for about 4 to 10 hours.

Yield: 4-servings

Nutritional values per serving: 386 Calories | 28.9g Fats | 6.4g Net Carbohydrates | 19.9g Protein

3. Spiced Pumpkin Puree

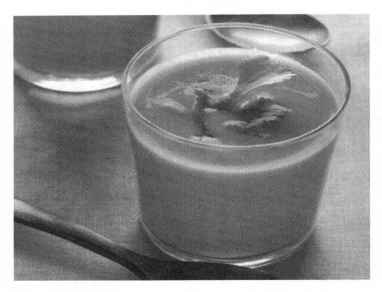

Ingredients:

1½-cups chicken broth

1-cup pumpkin puree

4-tbsps butter

4-slices bacon

3-tbsps bacon grease (from the bacon)

2-cloves garlic, minced, roasted

1-pc bay leaf

½-tsp salt

½-tsp pepper

½-tsp ginger, freshly minced

½-cup heavy cream

¼-tsp coriander

¼-tsp cinnamon

¼-bulb onion, medium, chopped

⅛-tsp nutmeg

Directions:

In a saucepan over medium-low heat, melt the butter until browned. Add onions, garlic, and ginger to the pan. Cook for about 2 to 3 minutes.

Add the spices when onions are translucent, and stir well. Cook for a couple of minutes, and then add pumpkin puree and chicken broth to the pan. Stir well.

Bring the mixture to a boil. Switch to low heat and allow simmering for about 20 minutes. Using an immersion blender, emulsify the broth mixture to a smooth consistency. Simmer for another 20 minutes.

In the meantime, cook the slices of bacon with its own grease until crisp. Set aside after cooking.

Add the bacon grease and heavy cream. Mix to combine well.

You may add chopped parsley and 2-tbsps of sour cream, as desired. Serve by crumbling the bacon over the broth.

Yield: 3 x 1-cup servings

Nutritional values per serving:

486 Calories | 48.7g Fats | 7.3g Net Carbohydrates | 5.7g Protein

Chapter 10 – Losing FATS; Gaining the BeneFITS

Work with the winning way to weigh less and wellness!

BeneFIT Fast from Feeding FATS!

Although the establishment of the ketogenic diet was initially for the exclusive treatment of epilepsy and other problems of the nervous system, more and more people have now favorably accepted to practice the diet with a variety of sensible reasons. Foremost of these reasons is its remarkable effect of shedding excessive weight while gaining more energy in the process.

More importantly, a host of other wellness benefits supports the diet's continued practice. From another standpoint, medical researchers worldwide continuously conduct extensive studies about the keto diet for more possible positive breakthroughs of treating and/or preventing other health neurological issues.

For the record, the European Journal of Clinical Nutrition compiled in June 2013 the following report about the different health conditions that ketogenic diets have been dealing with successfully:

Rapid Weight Reduction

Cutting down on carbohydrate is among the simplest, yet, most effective ways to lose weight. Studies will even show that individuals engaged in low-carbohydrate diets tend losing more weight much faster as compared to practitioners of low-fat diets (despite the fact that low-fat dieters keep on limiting calories aggressively)!

The principal reason behind such outcomes is that low-carbohydrate diets decrease the levels of insulin, which stimulates sodium retention. Moreover, such diets normally incur a diuretic effect that induces draining excess water from your body. In effect, your kidney will begin ridding out excess sodium that causes fluid or water retention and the creation of a temporary fluid weight gain.

Therefore, working with the diet directly results in faster weight reduction, even within a mere couple of weeks! Besides, bear in mind that under a ketogenic diet, your body is virtually a fat-burning machine!

Craving and Appetite Suppression

Practicing the ketogenic diet consequentially leads to automatic suppressions on your cravings and appetite. Thus, even without trying, you will frequently end up consuming much lesser calories. Resultant reductions in weight, needless to say, occur accordingly when levels of your appetites decline!

Metabolic Syndrome Treatments – The metabolic syndrome is an aggregation of the following symptoms:

- Low HDL Levels

- High LDL Levels

- High Triglycerides Levels

- High Blood Pressure Levels

- High Blood Sugar Levels

- Destructive Abdominal Fats Buildup or Obesity

Through the ketogenic diet, it effectively alters and reverses all the aforementioned symptoms, which often link to risks of heart disease and diabetes.

High-Density Lipoprotein (HDL) Cholesterol Level Enhancement

As a review of your lipoprotein functions, they are responsible for transporting cholesterols along the bloodstreams in your body. On the one hand, High-Density Lipoprotein (HDL) bears cholesterol away from the body and towards the liver, where it may excrete or reuse cholesterol. On the other hand, Low-Density Lipoprotein (LDL) moves cholesterol from the liver and towards the different parts of the body.

Since a keto diet is high in fat, it causes an impressive increase in blood levels of HDL, more known as the good cholesterol. However, a common indicator of heart disease risks is the HDL-triglycerides ratio. A higher ratio denotes greater risks of heart ailments. Ketogenic diets give rise to enhanced ratios by raising HDL levels while reducing triglycerides.

Low-Density Lipoprotein (LDL) Cholesterol Size Improvement

Individuals with high levels of LDL, notably known as the bad cholesterol, have higher tendencies of undergoing heart attacks. Nevertheless, what particularly counts the most is the LDL quality that corresponds to its particle sizes.

Further studies revealed that a keto diet improves the sizes of LDL particles from small to large. As it is the case, density wise, it simultaneously reduces the quantities of LDL particles in the bloodstream. People with mostly smaller LDL particles entail higher chances of heart ailments. Conversely, people with mostly larger particles obtain lower coronary disease risks.

Reduction of Triglycerides Levels

Triglycerides, which are fat molecules in the blood, are noted risk factors for heart diseases. The keto diet is more effective at drastically reducing blood triglycerides than a low-fat regimen, wherein, blood triglycerides have tendencies of shooting up in most cases.

Reduction of Blood Pressure Levels

Hypertension, or interchangeably known as high blood pressure, is a principal risk factor for several health problems such as heart disease, stroke, kidney failure, dementia or mental deterioration and more. Studies about the keto diet showed that lowering carbohydrate intakes causes a significant reduction in blood pressure. Thereby, the keto regimen, in effect, implies reduced risks of a myriad of common diseases.

Insulin and Blood Sugar Levels Reduction

Reducing the consumption of carbohydrates is the most efficient way to lower insulin and blood sugar levels. Furthermore, a low-carbohydrate intake is a very effective treatment method for insulin-resistant Type-2 diabetes mellitus with even higher possibilities of reversing the condition.

Nonetheless, if you intend reducing your blood sugar levels while currently under medication, then you must first consult with your doctor before devising any changes in your carbohydrate consumption. You may never know that your medication dosage might require certain adjustments to avoid hypoglycemia (glucose deficiency in the bloodstream).

Destructive Abdominal Fats Reduction

Fats differ relatively as to their stored locations in your body. These fat storage locations determine how they affect your health. They are either subcutaneous fats, stored under your skin, or visceral fats, stored in the abdominal cavity and prone to nestle in your different body organs. Prominent accumulations of visceral fats result in organ inflammation, insulin resistance, and metabolic dysfunction.

Keto diets become more effective at reducing all these fats dramatically, with larger percentages of fat loss occurring in the abdominal cavity. Practicing the diet over time, your body decreases its risks of acquiring heart diseases and Type 2 diabetes mellitus impressively.

Provisional Potencies

Advanced medical studies adjudged the ketogenic diet as an effective treatment for a wide variety of rare metabolic diseases. Some case reports even indicated the diet's potentiality for treating astrocytomas, which is a common type of primary brain tumor and found throughout the central nervous system. Other minor case studies concluded in unison that the diet improves worsening conditions of migraine headaches, type 2 diabetes mellitus, depression, autism, and polycystic ovary syndrome (PCOS).

Also, several clinical tests showed proofs that ketogenic diets cause favorable changes in the activity of disease symptoms encompassing neuro-degenerative conditions. Such nerve disorders include Parkinson's disease, Alzheimer's disease, and amyotrophic lateral sclerosis (ALS), also known as Lou Gehrig's disease or motor neuron disease, which is actually a breaking down of tissues in the nervous system.

Accounting for the fact that these aforementioned neuro-degenerative disorders impair the glucose metabolism of the brain, neurological studies bring up suggestions that ketone bodies produced in a state of ketosis offer to be alternative energy sources for the brain. Therefore, the overall treatment efficiencies of the ketogenic diet essentially serve as a protective mechanism in traumatic brain injuries, nervous system issues, and coronary heart diseases.

Therapy for Brain Disorders

While our brain significantly requires certain amounts of glucose, only a few brain components can burn glucose for energy conversion. Nevertheless, a greater part of our brain can easily burn ketone bodies as an alternative to glucose. Thus, the energy conversion function of your brain becomes more efficient when you undergo a keto diet.

Tumor cells produce energy and thrive by taking up glucose to burn at much higher rates than other cells. However, these cancer cells are inefficient at burning ketone bodies for energy. Eventually, they weaken and cease flourishing with ketones around and a low glucose supply. Therefore, medical experts believe that the ketogenic diet is also highly recommendable as possible effective benefits to brain cancer (such as glioma brain tumor) therapy.

Chapter 11 – Practical Program Pointers

A tight appetite is uptight!

The key to keto dieting is to curb a carb craving!

Although it may not be necessary tracking down your daily carbohydrate and calorie consumptions, it definitely helps to know precisely what you are consuming to point out easily your wrong steps along the way. It would be more beneficial learning a few tips and techniques towards your success in engaging with the ketogenic regimen:

1. Keep in mind the recommended and appropriate items for each food group. This will greatly facilitate you towards knowing what foods are suitably necessary for consumption and those you ought to avoid.

2. Learn about your macros or macronutrient consumptions. These intakes include the triumvirate of major nutrients— fats, proteins, and net carbohydrates, which denote your total dietary carbohydrate intake should be less tan your total fiber intake. Becoming aware of your macros allows you to measure or estimate the quantities of calories and nutrients you need to consume in order to reach your goals and achieve a successful practice of the ketogenic diet.

3. Bound yourself to become selective with your goals; only apply either a 10-15% calorie surplus or a 20-25% calorie deficit. According to studies, exceeding beyond the deficit values may incur undesirable effects concerning your dieting. Also, since the ketogenic diet is a perfect way of building up your muscles, you should know that protein intake is responsible for growing and strengthening your muscle tissues. Thus, when planning to gain muscular mass, you should consume about 1.0- 1.2g of protein per lean pound of your body weight.

4. Know your body activity levels. This will provide you a more realistic view about the normal quantities of calories that your body needs to burn daily.

5. Check and control! When finding yourself famished throughout your day, try curtailing your appetite by snacking on cheeses, peanut butter, seeds, and nuts. Snacks are integral in your meal plan, so they should also be under regulation.

Indeed, there is no real harm indulging with the ketogenic diet lest having a history of kidney health problems or Type-1 diabetes. Nevertheless, since your body is yet to adapt to the discipline, the first few days of the course of dieting normally gives you some lethargic moods and movements or severe headaches. Just allow getting the hang of it for a few weeks, especially during its initial hump; and definitely, you will eventually learn to curb your usual carb cravings!

Do's & Don'ts during Dine-outs

There are inevitable circumstances in our schedules that do not allow us to prepare our own food. Occasionally, we find ourselves dropping by at fast food outlets, attending parties, or dining out in fancy restaurants. These instances tend to derail you off the tracks of the ketogenic diet. There are those possibilities of consuming foods that you perceived as proper within the bounds of the keto regimen, but leave you clueless and unknowing about the surreptitious extent of carbohydrates composing your food.

Worry not, though. You may still be able to adhere to your keto meal plan and staying on course with your dietary program. The following are handy tips to help you out somehow in making the best out of the circumstances:

1. Bearing the primordial instinct of cutting down on your carbohydrates, know the dietary values and contents of your food.

2. As your alternatives for carbohydrates, choose salads and selected fruits.

3. Soy typically contains gluten, which is high in proteins; so, be sure you are not scanning a menu from a soy-based vegetarian diner.

4. Get into the habit of asking to check if the food served has hints of any sugar content. Better yet, verify the food's composition before ordering.

5. Choose eating places that allow you to feed substantially on seafood or meats. However, check their derived sources, whether or not the food comes from corn- or grain-fed livestock or, soy-fed sea produce.

6. Refrain from pastas and noodles derived from soy or whole-wheat grains.

7. Request for melted butter or olive oil to retain or attain your keto diet ratios.

8. Beware of sauces, salsas, and dressings. All of which may contain much sugar. Rather choose fast food chains serving salads with low-carbohydrate dressings.

9. Broiled or buttered is better than breaded or battered. Also, opt for a roasted, grilled, or baked food cooking process.

10. Hot dogs and hamburgers are fine, but irresistibly finer when eaten sans the buns. Wrap your burger or doggie with fresh lettuce leaves instead.

11. When hunger strikes while hitting the road, you can stuff your tummy with string cheese, hard-boiled eggs, deli meat, almonds, or pork rinds, or any other allowable keto snack items.

12. Order an espresso or double espresso for your coffee brew. Be it a Red Eye or Americano, a Sling Blade, Depth Charge or Turbo, include ordering almonds and either coconut milk or unsweetened heavy whipped cream for your creamer.

As with any type of dieting, the key to your success is preparing your food in advance, or simply, creating a meal plan. Having a definite guideline lets you stay focused while not veering away from your goals, as well as from the main objectives of the diet itself. Upon keeping your focus to begin a healthier, yet, more realistic approach of shedding body fat, you will truly realize with a smile that a keto diet and lifestyle is all worthwhile.

Alter your eating philosophies and lifestyles altogether... to alter your life for the better... forever!

Conclusion

Although the standard American diet (SAD) constitutes between 45% and 65% of calories acquired from carbohydrates, a ketogenic diet comparatively restricts the consumption of carbohydrates to a mere 2% to 4% of calories. Contrary to the beliefs of some people and many pseudo-experts, always note that the ketogenic diet is never a protein-rich regimen. Comparatively, a ketogenic diet emphasizes to compose foods rich in natural or organic fats and adequate proteins, and at the same time, a drastic limitation of foods high in carbohydrates.

The working principle of the diet is to attain ketosis in your body in order to avail ketone bodies as a substitute for carbohydrate-rich glucose during your body's energy conversion process. As glucose wanes and ketone bodies dominate along your bloodstreams, all of your major organs, including your muscles, brain, and heart ultimately discontinue burning glucose or sugar. Instead, these organs rely upon ketones and apply them as alternative fuel sources to energize your body; hence, establishing optimal or nutritional ketosis.

Such a consumption of more fats and regulated proteins and reduced carbohydrates results to changes in your metabolism. The changes produce more stored fats and ketone bodies for energy conversion; and thus, decreasing blood sugar levels, which is needless to say, a healthy and wellness sign for the body.

Aside from lowering blood sugar levels soon after the body attains optimal ketosis, a host of other beneficial outcomes ensue. First off, a high fat, low-carb, ketone-producing regimen works excellently in shedding your excess kilos. In turn, it allows you to stay fit and trim and thus raising your mood and energy levels. Consequently, it addresses an array of health issues that directly slows down your aging process.

In fact, compared to what other trendy and popular regimens may suggest, the ketogenic diet is greatly more effective. The anti-oxidant and anti-inflammatory effects brought about by optimal ketosis or by the conversion of chemically stable monounsaturated and saturated fats prove and manifest to be very powerful. Indeed, a ketogenic diet provides great impacts and benefits to your health.

In conclusion, the ketogenic diet is totally neither a passing trend nor a fad of the times. It is essentially a potent regulator of the body's metabolic disorders. With a proper implementation and practice, it exhausts all its capabilities of being extremely effective. The meat of the matter for ketogenic diets is all about how you can stay fit and trim, heighten your energy levels, and enhance your general health and welfare by simply altering the way you consume foods.

Made in the USA
San Bernardino, CA
15 May 2019